I0695558

Intermittent Fasting and Type 2 Diabetes in Women

Intermittent Fasting and Type 2 Diabetes in Women

What You
Need
to
Know

Jessie Asher

Dedication

This book is really dedicated to God for His grace and wisdom, my cherished family, the beautiful readers who will find connection inside these pages, and every amazing supporter who paved the way for me. You have led me to this point through your unwavering faith. All readers, especially diabetics, receive a renewal. This book is your travel buddy and your journey is important.

Table of Contents

Acknowledgement

I want to express my heartfelt thanks to God for guiding me throughout the creation of this book. My family's unwavering support and the invaluable contributions of my editor, publisher, and collaborators have shaped its success. To my friends, your constant encouragement has meant the world.

For the amazing picture, a special thanks to freepik.com and diabetesfoodhub.org.

Furthermore, I want to thank everyone who has read my work and appreciates it very much. I'm glad I got to experience it with you because it's been an amazing ride.

Introduction

Welcome to an exciting journey that promises to transform the way you think about health and diabetes management. Get ready to explore the intriguing world of intermittent fasting (IF), a dietary strategy that's not just a trend but a powerful tool for enhancing well-being. This book is your guide to understanding, embracing, and mastering intermittent fasting, especially tailored for women dealing with the growing concern of type 2 diabetes.

Understanding the Significance of Intermittent Fasting

Picture this: a dietary approach that not only helps you manage your weight but also rewires your body for better blood sugar control, improved metabolism, and overall health. That's the magic of intermittent fasting. But it's not a one-size-fits-all solution; it's a versatile strategy that requires a deep understanding of how it works and how to make it work for you.

Throughout this book, we'll delve into the nitty-gritty of intermittent fasting. You'll uncover the science behind it, explore the various fasting methods, and learn how to customize your fasting plan to suit your unique lifestyle and health goals.

The Growing Concern of Type 2 Diabetes in Women

Now, let's talk about a pressing issue: type 2 diabetes, a condition that's on the rise, especially among women. But here's the twist:

Women face a distinct set of challenges when it comes to managing diabetes. Hormonal fluctuations, life stage transitions like menopause, and diverse lifestyle factors all come into play. It's like solving a complex puzzle. In this book, we'll equip you with the knowledge and strategies you need to navigate these challenges effectively.

We're not just here to help you control your diabetes; we're here to support your overall wellbeing. In addition to including intermittent fasting as a potent weapon in your toolbox, we'll address the specific worries and inquiries women have regarding diabetes.

Purpose and Scope of this Book

So, what's our mission? Simply put, we aim to be your ultimate companion on your journey to managing type 2 diabetes with intermittent fasting. This isn't just another health book; it's your roadmap to a healthier and more empowered you.

Throughout these pages, we'll dive deep into the world of intermittent fasting, breaking down complex concepts into practical advice and actionable steps. We'll provide evidence-based insights, and offer personalized guidance. Our goal? To empower you with the knowledge and tools you need to make informed decisions about your health and well-being.

Are you ready to embark on this empowering journey? Together, we'll unravel the mysteries of intermittent fasting, tackle diabetes head-on, and empower you to take control of your health like never before. Get ready for a detailed exploration of intermittent fasting and diabetes management, tailored just for you. Let's get started!

Chapter 1

Type 2 Diabetes

Type 2 diabetes is a chronic condition that prevents your body from properly utilizing insulin. The most susceptible age group for this type of diabetes is middle age or older. Diabetes mellitus or adult-onset diabetes were the previous names for it. But because of childhood obesity, type 2 diabetes also affects children and adolescents.

With a significant impact on human life and healthcare costs, type 2 diabetes is acknowledged as a critical public health concern. In many regions of the world, the prevalence of diabetes is increasing due to rapid economic development and urbanization.

In 2017, there were around 462 million cases of type 2 diabetes worldwide, or 6.28% of the population (4.4% of people aged 15 to 49, 15% of people aged 50 to 69, and 22% of people aged 70 and older). This corresponds to a prevalence rate of 6059 cases per 100,000 people. Diabetes alone is responsible for almost 1 million fatalities annually, ranking it as the tenth most common cause of death.

By 2030, the global prevalence of type 2 diabetes is expected to climb to 7079 cases per 100,000 people, demonstrating an ongoing rise in all geographical areas.

Type 2 diabetes is more likely to occur in you if:

- You are Black, Hispanic, American Indian, Asian, Pacific Islander, or Asian American.
- You are over 45 years old.
- You are overweight or obese.
- You Don't work out (Exercise)
- You became pregnant while having gestational diabetes.
- You have diabetes running in your family.
- Your blood pressure is high.
- You have prediabetes (blood sugar levels that are higher than normal but not high enough to cause Type 2 diabetes).

A chronic metabolic illness called type 2 diabetes is characterized by high blood sugar (glucose) levels. It develops when your blood glucose, often known as blood sugar, is too high. Your body uses blood glucose as its primary energy source, which is primarily obtained from food.

The pancreas produces the hormone insulin, which facilitates the entry of glucose into cells for energy production. When you have type 2 diabetes, your body either produces insufficient insulin or uses it poorly. Thus, an excessive amount of glucose remains in the circulation while insufficient amounts reach your cells.

Causes of Type 2 Diabetes

Type 2 diabetes is a complex condition influenced by various factors. First and foremost, genetics plays a significant role. If you have close family members with type 2 diabetes, your risk goes up. Another key factor is obesity, especially excess weight around the abdomen, which can lead to insulin resistance, where your cells don't respond well to insulin.

Lifestyle choices matter too. Physical inactivity and a poor diet high in sugar and unhealthy fats contribute to the risk. Surprisingly, even if you're not overweight, your cells might become insulin resistant. Age is also a factor, with risk increasing after 45.

If you had gestational diabetes during pregnancy, you're more susceptible. Conditions like Polycystic Ovary Syndrome (PCOS), high blood pressure, and high cholesterol levels can also contribute. Smoking is associated with an increased risk, and even sleep apnea can make you more prone to insulin resistance. It's a multifaceted issue, but understanding these causes and risk factors is crucial for prevention and management.

While these factors can increase the risk, it's essential to note that type 2 diabetes can often be managed or prevented through lifestyle changes such as a healthy diet, regular exercise, and weight management, as well as medication or insulin therapy if prescribed by a healthcare professional.

Common signs and symptoms of type 2 diabetes

1. Increased thirst and hunger: You may experience excessive thirst and hunger, even after eating.
2. Frequent urination: You might need to urinate more frequently, especially at night.
3. Fatigue: Feeling unusually tired and lacking energy is common.
4. Blurred vision: High blood sugar levels can affect your vision.
5. Slow wound healing: Cuts and bruises may take longer to heal.
6. Tingling or numbness: Some individuals experience tingling or numbness in their hands or feet.
7. Recurrent infections: Type 2 diabetes can make you more susceptible to infections.
8. Weight changes: Unexplained weight loss or gain can occur.
9. Dark patches on the skin: Known as acanthosis nigricans, these are dark, velvety patches often found in body folds.

If you think you may have type 2 diabetes, you must see a doctor for an accurate diagnosis and treatment. Depending on the individual, these symptoms may or may not be present at all.

Type 2 diabetes can lead to various complications over time. Some common complications include:

- Cardiovascular Issues: Increased risk of heart disease, heart attacks, and stroke.

- Kidney Disease: Diabetes can damage the kidneys, potentially leading to kidney failure.

- Eye Problems: It can cause diabetic retinopathy, which may result in vision loss.

- Nerve Damage: Known as diabetic neuropathy, it can lead to numbness, tingling, and pain, often in the extremities.

- Foot Problems: Poor circulation and nerve damage can lead to foot ulcers and, in severe cases, amputation.

- Skin Conditions: Diabetes can cause skin issues, including infections and slow wound healing.

- Hypertension: High blood pressure is common among those with diabetes, increasing the risk of complications.

- Gastroparesis: Digestive problems can occur due to delayed stomach emptying.

- Depression: A higher risk of mental health issues, such as depression, is associated with diabetes.

- Alzheimer's Disease: Some studies suggest a link between diabetes and an increased risk of Alzheimer's.

Management and lifestyle changes, such as blood sugar control, a healthy diet, exercise, and medication, can help reduce the risk and severity of these complications. Regular medical check-ups are essential for early detection and intervention.

Diagnosis of Type 2 Diabetes

The diagnosis of type 2 diabetes typically involves several steps and medical tests. Here's an overview of how it's diagnosed:

1. *Medical History*: Your doctor will begin by asking about your medical history, including any symptoms you've been experiencing, family history of diabetes, and other relevant information.

2. *Physical Examination*: A physical examination may be conducted to check for signs of diabetes, such as high blood pressure, obesity, or skin changes.

3. *Fasting Blood Sugar Test*: This is one of the most common initial tests. You'll be asked to fast overnight (usually for 8 hours), and then a blood sample is taken to measure your fasting blood sugar level. A fasting blood sugar level of 126

milligrams per deciliter (mg/dL) or higher on two separate occasions is indicative of diabetes.

4. *Oral Glucose Tolerance Test* (OGTT): In some cases, an OGTT may be performed. You'll fast overnight, and then you'll drink a sugary solution. Blood sugar levels are tested at intervals over the next few hours. A blood sugar level of 200 mg/dL or higher two hours after drinking the solution may indicate diabetes.

5. *Hemoglobin A1c Test*: This test provides an average of your blood sugar levels over the past two to three months. An A1c level of 6.5% or higher is often used to diagnose diabetes.

6. *Random Blood Sugar Test*: In certain situations, a random blood sugar test may be done, especially if you have severe symptoms of high blood sugar. A result of 200 mg/dL or higher suggests diabetes.

7. *Glycated Albumin Test or Fructosamine Test*: These tests measure your average blood sugar levels over a shorter period, typically two to three weeks.

8. *Urine Tests*: Urine tests may be used to detect the presence of glucose or ketones in your urine, which can be a sign of uncontrolled diabetes.

9. *Additional Tests*: Depending on your specific situation, your healthcare provider may recommend additional tests

to evaluate your overall health and any potential complications associated with diabetes.

Management of Type 2 Diabetes

Changes in lifestyle, medication (if ordered by a healthcare provider), and routine blood sugar monitoring are all part of managing type 2 diabetes.

Here are key aspects of type 2 diabetes management:

1. Healthy Eating
- Follow a balanced diet that includes a variety of foods, focusing on vegetables, fruits, whole grains, lean proteins, and healthy fats.
- Monitor carbohydrate intake and distribute it evenly throughout the day to help regulate blood sugar levels.
- Limit sugary and highly processed foods and beverages.

2. Regular Physical Activity
- Aim for at least 150 minutes of moderate-intensity aerobic exercise per week, such as brisk walking or cycling.
- Include strength training exercises at least two days a week.
- Exercise helps improve insulin sensitivity and can help control blood sugar.

3. Weight Management
- Achieving and maintaining a healthy weight can significantly improve blood sugar control.

- If overweight, losing even a small amount of weight (5-10% of your body weight) can make a significant difference.

4. Medication

- Some people with type 2 diabetes may require medication or insulin therapy prescribed by a healthcare provider.
- Medications can help lower blood sugar levels and may include oral medications or injectable insulin.

5. Blood Sugar Monitoring

- Regularly check your blood sugar levels as advised by your healthcare team.
- Keep a record of your readings to identify patterns and make necessary adjustments to your treatment plan.

6. Stress Management

High stress levels can affect blood sugar.

- Practice stress-reduction techniques such as deep breathing, meditation, or yoga.

7. Regular Healthcare Checkups

- Schedule regular checkups with your healthcare provider to monitor your overall health and diabetes management.
- Address any concerns or questions you have about your condition.

8. Foot Care

- Check your feet daily for cuts, sores, or signs of infection, and report any issues to your healthcare provider.

- Proper foot care is crucial to prevent diabetes-related foot problems.

9. Education and Support
- Learn about diabetes and how to manage it effectively through education programs or support groups.
- Involve family and friends in your diabetes management to create a supportive environment.

10. Medication Adherence

If a medicine is prescribed, follow the instructions provided by your doctor and talk to them about any adverse effects or concerns you may have.

11. Blood Pressure and Cholesterol Control

Manage your blood pressure and cholesterol levels to reduce the risk of cardiovascular complications, which are common in people with diabetes.

The management of type 2 diabetes is individualized, and your healthcare team will work with you to create a personalized plan that satisfies your unique requirements and objectives. Effectively controlling type 2 diabetes and lowering the risk of complications requires consistent self-care and regular communication with your healthcare professional.

Chapter 2

Exploring Type 2 Diabetes in Women

Despite the fact that diabetes affects men more frequently than women, according to the Centers for Disease Control and Prevention (CDC), women are said to be more vulnerable to complications and hazards after a diagnosis. Though type 2 diabetes can lead to serious complications in women, such as heart disease and issues with fertility, early diagnosis and blood sugar management are essential for avoiding serious health issues.

Type 2 diabetes can strike anyone at any age, however two groups of women are at higher risk than others:
- those over 45
- those who are obese or overweight.

Although type 2 diabetes mellitus is more common in both sexes, males are often diagnosed earlier and have lower body fat mass than women. In the world, men are predicted to have diabetes mellitus in 17.7 million more people than women. When type 2 diabetes is diagnosed, women seem to have a heavier burden of risk factors, especially obesity. In addition, women may be more at risk for diabetes due to psychosocial stress.

Women are more prone than males to develop depression if they have type 2 diabetes. The severity and frequency of type 2 diabetes complications are influenced by depression. In a study published in 2020, depression was linked to a more than 50% higher chance of type 2 diabetes-related hospitalizations.

Women's sexual health is impacted by type 2 diabetes as well. In a 2015 study, more than 78% of type 2 diabetic women reported experiencing some form of sexual dysfunction, including:

- Vaginal dryness, which can make sex difficult or uncomfortable
- less sex drive
- Difficulties achieving orgasm or sexual arousal
- low level of sex enjoyment

Impaired estrogen signaling brought on by elevated blood sugar levels may possibly be a contributing factor in these issues. It could get worse during menopause, when changes in hormone levels have an effect on vaginal dryness and sexual function. In women with uncontrolled type 2 diabetes, high blood sugar can further raise the risk of pregnancy-related problems, including the risk of:

- Preeclampsia or high blood pressure
- Cesarean section
- a stillbirth or miscarriage.

Anyone with type 2 diabetes who is expecting a baby or who intends to conceive should work closely with their medical team to keep their blood sugar levels under control.

Type 2 diabetes has become more common over time, and this trend is predicted to continue. When possible, recognizing potential risk factors for diabetes enables medical professionals to diagnose the condition earlier or suggest modifications for prevention.

According to a survey, there are over 199 million diabetic women worldwide. Furthermore, it is anticipated that this would reach 313 million by 2040. It is also the ninth most prevalent cause of death for women globally, accounting for 2.1 million annual fatalities, many of which are preventable.

In reality, the study discovered that women:

- have a four-fold increased risk of cardiovascular illness as a result of diabetes

- are more likely than men to experience various health issues like depression, kidney disease, and blindness.

- If they plan to become pregnant while having diabetes or are at a high risk of developing it, they should seriously evaluate their options.

Diabetes currently affects 415 million people worldwide; by 2040, that number is expected to rise to almost half a billion. 90–95% of

the 37 million Americans who have the disease are type 2
diabetics.

In England, it is estimated that 3.8 million adults (16 and older)
have diabetes, both diagnosed and undiagnosed. This equates to
8.6% of the total number of people in this age group. Men are more
likely than women to have diabetes (9.6% vs. 7.6%).

Risk Factors

The following are typical risk factors that have been closely linked
to type 2 diabetes, according to one academic review:

- Type 2 diabetes and diabetes in the family history
- Obesity
- High serum uric acid levels
- Smoking
- Depression
- Dyslipidemia
- Hypertension
- Cardiovascular disease
- Aging
- Quantity and quality of sleep
- Ethnicity (including Pacific Islanders, African Americans, Asian Americans, and Native Americans from the United States, Alaska, and Hawaii)

However, several studies have indicated that sex-specific risk factors can exist. For instance, according to one study, women are more likely than males to be affected by these two risk factors:

- High amounts of uric acid and being inactive physically.

In addition, women are more likely to be diagnosed with type 2 diabetes if they have a history of:

- Gestational diabetes mellitus (GDM or GD):

Type 2 diabetes is more likely to develop in pregnant women with gestational diabetes (GD).

- Polycystic ovary syndrome (PCOS):

One investigation found a connection between PCOS and type 2 diabetes' insulin resistance.

Gender-Specific Challenges

Of course, type 2 diabetes has issues that are specific to certain genders as well. It's important to note that these challenges can vary widely among individuals, and diabetes management should be personalized to each person's unique needs and circumstances.

Challenges for Men

1. Lower Awareness: Men may be less likely to recognize the early signs of diabetes and seek medical attention.

2. Reluctance to Seek Help: Men, in general, might be less inclined to visit healthcare professionals regularly, delaying diabetes management.

3. Risky Behaviors: Certain male behaviors like higher rates of smoking and alcohol consumption can exacerbate diabetes-related complications.

Challenges for Women

1. Hormonal Fluctuations: Women experience hormonal changes during their menstrual cycle, pregnancy, and menopause, which can affect blood sugar levels and require specific management.

2. Stereotypes and Body Image: Societal pressures related to body image and weight can affect women's self-esteem and their approach to diabetes management.

3. Gestational Diabetes: Pregnant women may develop gestational diabetes, which can affect both mother and baby's health.

4. Polycystic Ovary Syndrome (PCOS): PCOS is more common in women with type 2 diabetes and can complicate diabetes management.

5. Social and Cultural Factors: Gender roles and expectations can influence diabetes management and access to healthcare.

6. Cardiovascular Risk: Women with diabetes face a higher risk of heart disease than men with diabetes.

7. Depression and Eating Disorders: These conditions are more prevalent in women with type 2 diabetes and can impact diabetes management.

8. Access to Care: Socioeconomic factors can affect women's access to healthcare, medication, and education about diabetes.

9. Pregnancy Planning: Women with diabetes need specialized care when planning for pregnancy to ensure a healthy pregnancy and baby.

These challenges highlight the importance of tailored healthcare approaches for individuals with type 2 diabetes based on their gender.

Impact on Women's Health

Type 2 diabetes can have a significant impact on women's health in several ways:

1. Hormonal Changes: Diabetes can affect hormonal balance, potentially leading to irregular menstrual cycles, polycystic ovary syndrome (PCOS), and fertility issues.

2. Gestational Diabetes: Some women develop gestational diabetes during pregnancy, which can increase the risk of complications for both the mother and the baby.

3. Increased Risk of Heart Disease: Women with type 2 diabetes have a higher risk of heart disease compared to women without diabetes.

4. Complications during Pregnancy: Uncontrolled diabetes during pregnancy can lead to birth complications, including macrosomia (large birth weight), preterm birth, and cesarean section.

5. Bladder and Kidney Problems: Diabetes can increase the risk of urinary tract infections and kidney problems, which can be more common in women.

6. Bone Health: Women with diabetes may have an increased risk of osteoporosis, leading to weaker bones.

7. Sexual Health: Diabetes can affect sexual function and lead to issues like vaginal dryness or decreased libido.

8. Mental Health: Managing diabetes can be emotionally challenging and may contribute to stress, anxiety, or depression in women.

9. Increased Risk of Infections: Women with diabetes may be more susceptible to certain infections, such as yeast infections.

10. Eye Health: Diabetes can increase the risk of diabetic retinopathy, which can lead to vision problems or blindness.

11. Neuropathy: Nerve damage (neuropathy) is a common complication of diabetes and can affect various parts of the body, including the feet and hands.

12. Long-Term Complications: Over time, uncontrolled diabetes can lead to severe complications such as kidney disease, peripheral artery disease, and stroke, all of which can impact women's health.

Proactive management of type 2 diabetes through lifestyle changes, medication, and regular medical check-ups is crucial for minimizing these health risks. Women with diabetes should work closely with their healthcare providers to develop a personalized diabetes management plan that addresses their unique needs.

Chapter 3

Intermittent Fasting

What Is Intermittent Fasting?

One of the most appreciated health and fitness fads nowadays is intermittent fasting (IF). Numerous studies demonstrate that it can have strong impacts on your body and brain and may even lengthen your life, and as such a lot of people use it to simplify their lives, lose weight, and enhance their health.

Intermittent fasting can be defined as an eating pattern that alternates between eating and fasting intervals. It's like a rhythm for when you eat, it's not about what you eat but when you eat. You have periods where you don't eat (fasting) and periods when you do (eating). Imagine skipping breakfast and only having lunch and dinner. That's a simple form of intermittent fasting. It's like giving your body a break from food for a while.

People do it for different reasons - some for weight loss, others for health benefits. It's kind of like telling your body, "Hey, let's take a pause from eating for a bit and see how it feels." Although it might have health advantages, including enhanced insulin sensitivity and weight management, it's crucial to speak with a doctor before beginning any fasting plan.

Fasting has been a habit for humans from the beginning of time. There were no supermarkets, refrigerators, or year-round food supplies available to early hunter-gatherers. They occasionally had trouble finding something to eat. As a result, humans have developed to be able to survive for extended periods of time without eating.

In actuality, intermittent fasting is more natural than consuming 3–4 (or more) meals per day. But remember, it's not a strict diet. You can adjust it to fit your lifestyle, and it's important to stay healthy and listen to your body while doing it.

Different Approaches to Intermittent Fasting

Intermittent fasting can be done in a variety of ways, each with unique fasting and eating times.

- 16/8 Method

This involves fasting for 16 hours a day and restricting your eating to an 8-hour window. For instance, you might eat from 12:00 PM to 8:00 PM and fast from 8:00 PM to 12:00 PM the next day.

- 5:2 Method

With this approach, you eat normally for five days of the week and consume very few calories (around 500-600) on the other two non-consecutive days.

- Eat-Stop-Eat

In this approach, you fast once or twice every week for a full 24 hours. For instance, you might fast between supper on one day and dinner on the following day.

- Alternate-Day Fasting

This involves alternating between fasting days and regular eating days. On fasting days, you consume very few calories or none at all.

- Warrior Diet

With this approach, you fast for 20 hours and have a 4-hour eating window typically in the evening. During the fasting hours, small amounts of raw fruits and vegetables may be consumed.

- OMAD (One Meal a Day)

In this approach, you only have one substantial meal every day, and the other 23 hours are spent fasting.

- The 36-Hour Fast

This involves fasting for a full 36 hours once or twice a week. For example, you might fast from breakfast one day until dinner the next day.

- Extended Fasting

Extended fasts can last several days or even weeks. They require careful planning, supervision, and may be best suited for experienced fasters or those with specific health goals.

- Circadian Rhythm Fasting

This approach aligns fasting with your body's natural circadian rhythms. It typically involves fasting during nighttime hours and eating during daylight hours, which can promote better sleep and metabolic health.

- Intermittent Fasting with Breakfast

If you prefer breakfast, you can have an early eating window, like 7 AM to 3 PM, and then fast until the next morning.

- Customized Schedules

You can create a fasting schedule that suits your unique needs, such as fasting on specific days of the week or adjusting eating windows to fit your routine.

It's critical to select the intermittent fasting strategy that best fits your way of life and health objectives. Additionally, it is wise to speak with a healthcare provider before beginning any fasting regimen, particularly if you have underlying medical issues.

How It Affects the Body

The body can be affected by intermittent fasting in a number of ways, both immediately and over time. Here are some effects it might have on your body:

1. *Weight Loss*: Intermittent fasting can help reduce calorie intake, leading to weight loss. During the fasting period, your body uses stored fat for energy.

2. *Improved Insulin Sensitivity*: By improving insulin sensitivity, intermittent fasting can increase the responsiveness of your cells to insulin. In order to assist move glucose (sugar) from the bloodstream into cells for energy, your body releases insulin when you consume, especially when it comes to carbohydrates. With increased sensitivity, your body uses less insulin to properly control blood sugar levels.

3. *Lower Insulin Levels*: Insulin levels sharply decline when people fast. This is advantageous as insulin resistance, a precursor to type 2 diabetes, can result from persistently elevated insulin levels. Better blood sugar regulation is encouraged by lower insulin levels. For instance, a small study indicated that IF reduced insulin resistance in 13 persons with type 2 diabetes. It was published in the journal Hormone and Metabolic Research in August 2021.

4. *Cellular Repair*: Fasting triggers a cellular process called autophagy, where cells remove damaged components. This can have potential benefits for longevity and disease prevention.

5. *Heart Health*: Some studies suggest that intermittent fasting can improve heart health by reducing risk factors

like high blood pressure, cholesterol levels, and inflammation.

6. *Brain Health*: Fasting may stimulate the production of brain-derived neurotrophic factor (BDNF), which is linked to improved brain function and a reduced risk of neurodegenerative diseases.

7. *Hormone Regulation*: Fasting can affect the release of hormones like ghrelin and leptin, which regulate hunger and fullness, potentially aiding in appetite control.

8. *Stress Resistance*: Fasting may enhance the body's ability to cope with stress and increase the production of stress resistance proteins.

9. *Stabilized Blood Sugar*: By preventing the spikes and crashes that might be brought on by frequent meals and snacks, intermittent fasting can help maintain blood sugar levels. Improved energy levels and general health may result from this blood sugar profile stabilization.

10. *Enhanced Fat Utilization*: During fasting, your body shifts from using glucose as its primary energy source to using stored fat. This can help reduce the accumulation of fat in the liver and muscles, which can contribute to insulin resistance.

It's important to understand that not everyone who practices intermittent fasting will experience the same advantages. Fasting should also be done safely and with consideration for each person's medical needs. Before beginning any fasting regimen, it is advised to speak with a healthcare provider, especially if you have underlying medical issues.

Chapter 4

Intermittent Fasting and Blood Sugar Regulation

"Intermittent Fasting and Blood Sugar Regulation" is all about how taking breaks from eating at certain times can help control your blood sugar levels. It's like giving your body a rest from food now and then. When you do this, your body uses up stored sugar for energy, which can lower your blood sugar. Plus, it can make your cells better at handling sugar, so your blood sugar stays in a healthy range. It's a bit like giving your body a tune-up to keep your blood sugar in check!

Fasting and Glucose Levels

The length and kind of fasting can both have an effect on how directly fasting affects the body's glucose levels. Fasting needs to be done carefully, especially if you have diabetes or other disorders that affect how your blood sugar is regulated.

Here's how fasting can affect glucose levels:

- Short-Term Fasting (Intermittent Fasting)

Fasting over a brief period of time, such as intermittent fasting, frequently causes a transient drop in blood sugar levels. The body uses glucose (glycogen) stored in the body during fasting periods, especially after several hours without eating. Blood glucose levels tend to drop as glycogen stores are used up. This can be especially useful for people trying to increase their insulin sensitivity.

- Prolonged Fasting

The body may begin converting stored fat into ketones for energy if a fast lasts for a long time, usually longer than 24 hours. Glucose can be substituted by ketones as a fuel source. Further drops in blood glucose levels may result from this. However, to avoid hypoglycemia (low blood sugar), it's crucial to monitor blood sugar levels throughout a prolonged fast, especially if you have diabetes.

- Post-Fasting Rebound

Blood glucose levels may increase after breaking a fast when the body starts to break down and absorb nutrients from the subsequent meal. If the meal contains a lot of carbohydrates, the blood sugar bounce that occurs after a fast may be more noticeable.

Before beginning any fasting regimen, speak with a medical professional to make sure it's secure for your particular circumstance. You may better understand how your body reacts by keeping an eye on your blood sugar levels both during and after meals. If necessary, you can then modify your fasting schedule accordingly.

How receptive your cells are to insulin is referred to as insulin sensitivity. You can lower your risk of numerous diseases, including diabetes, and insulin resistance by improving it. Your blood sugar levels are regulated by the hormone insulin, which is necessary. There is a link between insulin sensitivity and insulin resistance, you have poor insulin sensitivity if you have insulin resistance. Contrarily, if you have low insulin resistance, you have high insulin sensitivity. Increased insulin sensitivity is helpful for your health, however insulin resistance is detrimental.

Insulin sensitivity in women, like in men, plays a crucial role in overall metabolic health. Here are some key points regarding insulin sensitivity in women:

1. Hormonal Influence

Hormones like estrogen and progesterone can indeed influence insulin sensitivity in women, and these hormonal fluctuations can lead to variations in insulin sensitivity throughout the menstrual cycle.

During the luteal phase (the second half of the menstrual cycle), which occurs after ovulation and before menstruation, progesterone levels rise while estrogen levels may fluctuate. This hormonal shift can result in reduced insulin sensitivity and higher insulin resistance for some women during this phase. As a result, they may be more prone to experiencing slightly elevated blood sugar levels or changes in carbohydrate metabolism during this time.

These hormonal fluctuations are a natural part of a woman's menstrual cycle, and they can affect how the body responds to insulin. It's important for women to be aware of these variations, especially if they have underlying insulin resistance or diabetes, as they may need to adjust their diet, exercise, or medication management accordingly.

Maintaining a healthy lifestyle with a balanced diet and regular physical activity can help mitigate the effects of hormonal changes on insulin sensitivity throughout the menstrual cycle. If there are concerns about managing blood sugar levels during different phases of the menstrual cycle, consulting with a healthcare provider can provide tailored guidance and recommendations.

2. Pregnancy

During pregnancy, significant changes in insulin sensitivity occur as part of the body's natural adaptation to support the developing fetus and ensure a stable supply of glucose. Here's how insulin sensitivity changes during pregnancy:

- Early Pregnancy: In the first trimester, insulin sensitivity typically decreases. This temporary decrease in insulin sensitivity is thought to ensure that more glucose is available for the growing embryo and fetus. It helps divert glucose from the mother's cells to the developing placenta.

- Mid-to-Late Pregnancy: As pregnancy progresses, especially into the second and third trimesters, insulin resistance in the mother's body increases. This insulin resistance is essential for maintaining a higher blood glucose level, ensuring that the developing baby receives the necessary nutrients and energy.

- Gestational Diabetes: Some women experience a more pronounced increase in insulin resistance during pregnancy, leading to gestational diabetes. This condition can develop in the second half of pregnancy when the body's insulin production may not keep up with the rising insulin resistance, resulting in elevated blood sugar levels.

Pregnant women should periodically check their blood sugar levels, especially if they have risk factors for gestational diabetes, such as obesity or a family history of diabetes. To control blood sugar levels throughout pregnancy and protect the health of both the mother and the growing child, medical professionals may advise dietary changes, physical activity, and, in certain situations, insulin therapy.

Most women experience a return to pre-pregnancy levels of insulin sensitivity following delivery, while others may still have impaired glucose metabolism and need to be closely monitored.

3. Polycystic Ovary Syndrome (PCOS)

Polycystic Ovary Syndrome (PCOS) is a common hormonal disorder in women that is often associated with insulin resistance, and this increases the risk of type 2 diabetes and high blood sugar levels.

Here are some key points regarding PCOS and insulin sensitivity:

- Insulin Resistance: Many women with PCOS experience insulin resistance, where their cells don't respond effectively to insulin's signals. This leads to elevated insulin levels in an attempt to compensate for the reduced sensitivity of cells to insulin.

- Hormonal Imbalances: PCOS is characterized by hormonal imbalances, including high levels of androgens (male hormones) and irregular menstrual cycles. These hormonal disturbances can contribute to insulin resistance.

- Metabolic Complications: Insulin resistance in PCOS can increase the risk of several metabolic complications, including type 2 diabetes, obesity, and cardiovascular problems.

Working closely with healthcare professionals who can offer individualized advice and treatment programs catered to their particular needs is vital for women with PCOS. Addressing the different health issues related to PCOS requires managing insulin sensitivity by lifestyle adjustments and, if required, medications.

4. Menopause

Hormonal changes during menopause can significantly impact insulin sensitivity in women. Menopause is characterized by the cessation of menstruation and a decline in the production of estrogen and progesterone. These hormonal changes can lead to increased insulin resistance in some women, contributing to various health concerns:

- Weight Gain: Insulin resistance can make it easier to gain weight, particularly around the abdomen, which is a common concern for many women going through menopause.

- Metabolic Changes: The reduction in estrogen levels can affect metabolism, potentially leading to alterations in carbohydrate metabolism and an increased risk of elevated blood sugar levels.

- Risk of Type 2 Diabetes: The combination of increased insulin resistance and metabolic changes can raise the risk of developing type 2 diabetes during and after menopause.

- Cardiovascular Health: Insulin resistance is associated with an increased risk of cardiovascular disease, which can become a greater concern for postmenopausal women.

- Bone Health: Hormonal changes during menopause also impact bone health. Insulin resistance may affect bone metabolism, potentially influencing the risk of osteoporosis.

During and after menopause, women need to manage their insulin sensitivity. Improved insulin sensitivity can be attributed to lifestyle factors including maintaining a healthy weight through diet and exercise. In addition, some medical professionals could think about using hormone replacement therapy (HRT) to treat menopause symptoms, which might have an impact on how sensitive the body is to insulin. In order to create a customized plan for controlling insulin sensitivity and overall health, it's critical for women at this stage of life to talk with their healthcare professionals about their specific health needs and concerns.

5. Lifestyle Factors

Lifestyle factors, including diet, physical activity, and body composition, play a pivotal role in influencing insulin sensitivity for both women and men. Here's how these factors can impact insulin sensitivity:

- Diet: A balanced diet that includes a variety of nutrient-dense foods can help improve insulin sensitivity.

Key dietary considerations include:
  - Reducing the consumption of sugary foods and drinks.
  - Choosing complex carbohydrates (whole grains, fruits, vegetables) over simple sugars.
  - Incorporating lean protein sources.
  - Including healthy fats, such as those from avocados, nuts, and olive oil.

- Monitoring portion sizes to manage calorie intake.

- Physical Activity: Regular physical activity is one of the most effective ways to enhance insulin sensitivity. Exercise helps muscles take up glucose from the bloodstream more efficiently. Aerobic exercises like walking, running, and cycling, as well as resistance training, can be beneficial. Even small amounts of exercise, such as daily walking, can have a positive impact.

- Body Composition: Maintaining a healthy body weight and composition is crucial for insulin sensitivity. Excess body fat, particularly around the abdomen, is associated with increased insulin resistance. Achieving and maintaining a healthy weight through a combination of diet and exercise can help improve insulin sensitivity.

- Stress Management: Chronic stress can negatively affect insulin sensitivity. Practicing stress-reduction techniques such as mindfulness, meditation, and relaxation exercises can be beneficial.

- Adequate Sleep: Getting enough quality sleep is essential for metabolic health, including insulin sensitivity. Aim for 7-9 hours of restful sleep per night.

- Hydration: Staying well-hydrated is also important for metabolic health. Water helps regulate blood sugar levels, so it's essential to drink enough throughout the day.

- Meal Timing: Some research suggests that meal timing, such as spacing meals evenly throughout the day or practicing intermittent fasting, may also influence insulin sensitivity for some individuals. However, individual responses can vary.

6. Gestational Diabetes

Gestational diabetes can affect insulin sensitivity during pregnancy. Here's how it impacts insulin sensitivity:

- Insulin Resistance: Gestational diabetes is characterized by increased insulin resistance, where the body's cells become less responsive to insulin's effects. This insulin resistance develops as a natural adaptation during pregnancy to ensure that more glucose is available for the growing fetus.

- Increased Insulin Production: In response to insulin resistance, the pancreas typically produces more insulin to help maintain normal blood sugar levels. This can lead to higher-than-usual insulin levels in the bloodstream.

- Impaired Blood Sugar Regulation: Despite increased insulin production, some women with gestational diabetes may not produce enough insulin to overcome the resistance fully. This can result in elevated blood sugar levels, known as hyperglycemia, which can have health implications for both the mother and the baby.

- Effects on Insulin Sensitivity: During pregnancy, gestational diabetes largely impairs insulin sensitivity, which makes insulin less efficient at decreasing blood sugar levels. In order to reduce blood sugar levels and lessen the influence on insulin sensitivity, proper management is crucial. This may involve dietary adjustments, physical activity, and in some cases, medication or insulin therapy.

- Postpartum Changes: In many cases, insulin sensitivity returns to normal after childbirth. However, women who've had gestational diabetes should continue to monitor their blood sugar levels postpartum and maintain a healthy lifestyle to reduce the risk of developing type 2 diabetes later in life.

Effective gestational diabetes management is essential to avoiding problems and preserving the health of both the mother and the fetus. In order to help pregnant women manage their blood sugar levels and insulin sensitivity, healthcare professionals collaborate closely with them.

7. Individual Variability

Of course, depending on a variety of unique circumstances, women's reactions to insulin sensitivity can differ dramatically from men's depending on a variety of factors. A few important causes of this unpredictability are listed below:

- Genetics: Genetic factors can play a significant role in determining an individual's insulin sensitivity. Some people may have a genetic predisposition to be more insulin-sensitive, while others may have a genetic predisposition to be more insulin-resistant.

- Age: Insulin sensitivity tends to decline with age. Older individuals often experience reduced insulin sensitivity compared to younger ones.

- Body Composition: Body composition, particularly the amount of muscle mass versus fat, can influence insulin sensitivity. Lean muscle tissue tends to be more insulin-sensitive than fat tissue.

- Physical Activity: Regular physical activity can improve insulin sensitivity. Individuals who engage in consistent exercise often have better insulin sensitivity compared to those who are sedentary.

- Diet: Diet plays a significant role in insulin sensitivity. Consuming a diet high in refined sugars and processed carbohydrates can contribute to insulin resistance, while a balanced diet rich in whole foods can enhance sensitivity.

- Hormonal Factors: As discussed earlier, hormonal changes related to menstrual cycles, pregnancy, menopause, and conditions like polycystic ovary syndrome (PCOS) can influence insulin sensitivity in women.

- Medications and Health Conditions: Certain medications, such as corticosteroids or antipsychotic drugs, can affect insulin sensitivity. Health conditions like diabetes, obesity, and metabolic disorders also impact insulin sensitivity.

- Stress: Chronic stress can contribute to insulin resistance and negatively affect insulin sensitivity.

Women should be aware of their insulin sensitivity, especially if they have diabetes or other risk factors for insulin resistance. Maintaining a healthy lifestyle and routinely checking blood sugar levels can help control and enhance insulin sensitivity. Consulting with a healthcare professional can offer individualized advice and recommendations if you have questions regarding your insulin sensitivity or blood sugar control.

Chapter 5

Practical Intermittent Fasting Strategies

Practical Intermittent Fasting Strategies are like the secret tricks and tips for making your 'food timing' game strong! It's all about when you eat, not what you eat. Think of it as your personalized fasting schedule. It's like having a food clock. You choose when to start and stop eating during the day.

Picture this: you might decide to skip breakfast and have a later lunch, or maybe you're the type who skips dinner instead. That's your strategy, right there! These strategies help you make intermittent fasting work for your lifestyle. They keep you on track, keep you hydrated, and make sure you're not starving yourself. It's like your own tailor-made plan for healthier eating patterns. Cool, right?

Choosing the Right Fasting Schedule

Choosing the right fasting protocol means doing what's best for you. Here are three criteria to consider:

1. Ease

It should not be difficult to practice intermittent fasting. During your fasts, you should feel largely at ease. Despite this, you might still get hungry. We will always be hungry. You might want to halt and think twice, though, if the discomfort extends beyond hunger.

Here are some indications that your fasting protocol may require modification:

- You're having trouble sleeping
- When you're fasting, you're not in the best of moods.
- Your level of fitness has declined
- You experience weakness, fatigue, or stress.
- You dislike it when loved ones or friends eat in front of you.

Think about cutting back to a shorter fast if you exhibit one or more of these symptoms. It is worthwhile for your comfort and well-being.

2. Schedule

Your schedule will determine how long you fast. Alternate-day fasting might not be for you if your family observes a special mealtime custom. There may be a preference for family time. Make sure that your fasting schedule won't interfere too much with your ability to attend work meetings, social events, and family dinners.

However, generally speaking, fasting allows you more time. You may fill those blocks with other activities when you aren't stressed about preparing or eating meals. To increase productivity, many people, for instance, forgo breakfast. When dinner finally arrives, eating is seen as a reward for a job well done. Select a schedule that fits your daily routine.

If you have a consistent daily schedule, the 16/8 method might work well. If your days vary, consider flexible options like 5:2 or alternate-day fasting. Plan your eating and fasting times to coincide with your sleep cycles. You could discover that fasting at night is more pleasant.

3. Health goals

Why do you intend to fast? Is it to lose weight or to maintain a strong, slim body, or is it for additional health advantages?

Before deciding on a fasting schedule, be sure of this cause. The longer routines are likely more successful if your goal is to reduce weight. Your calorie intake will decrease as your meal window gets smaller. Nevertheless, bear in mind the ease requirement from criterion #1. You won't likely follow the plan if fasting is constantly uncomfortable for you.

The fact that prolonged fasts are not recommended for retaining or growing muscle is also crucial to understand. There is too much possibility for protein and calorie limitation. However, numerous studies have revealed that people can maintain muscle while resistance exercising on a 16/8 schedule. If strength development and muscle maintenance are your primary objectives, sixteen hours might be a fair upper limit.

For diabetics, working with your doctor will help you determine which schedule is best for you.

Combining Fasting with a Balanced Diet

For some people, combining a balanced diet and fasting can be a smart move. Here are some efficient and safe methods:

1. Intermittent Fasting (IF): Choose a fasting window (e.g., 16/8, 18/6) where you fast for a set number of hours each day. During your eating window, focus on consuming nutrient-dense foods.

2. Time Your Meals: Plan your meals around your fasting schedule. Prioritize whole grains, lean proteins, fruits, and vegetables to ensure balanced nutrition.

3. Don't forget Hydration: Stay hydrated, even during fasting periods. Water, herbal tea, or black coffee can be consumed without breaking the fast.

4. Protein Intake: Ensure you get enough protein to support muscle maintenance and overall health. Include lean meats, fish, tofu, or plant-based protein sources.

5. Variety of Foods: Incorporate a wide variety of foods to cover all essential nutrients. Include colorful fruits and vegetables, nuts, seeds, and whole grains.

6. Control Portions: Be mindful of portion sizes to avoid overeating when breaking your fast. Smaller, balanced meals are ideal.

7. Limit Processed Foods: Minimize processed and sugary foods, even during your eating window, as they can disrupt blood sugar levels.

8. Healthy Fats: Include sources of healthy fats like avocados, nuts, and olive oil to support satiety and overall health.

9. Plan Ahead: Prepare meals and snacks in advance to avoid reaching for unhealthy options when hunger strikes.

10. Consult a Professional: If you have underlying health conditions or specific dietary needs, consult a healthcare provider or registered dietitian before starting any fasting regimen.

Keep in mind that every person's needs are different, making fasting not ideal for everyone. To maintain a balanced and sustainable approach to mixing fasting with a nutritious diet, it's imperative to pay attention to your body, check your health, and make modifications as needed.

For women with type 2 diabetes, intermittent fasting may be advantageous, although caution is required.

Here are some pointers for long-term achievement:

1. *Consult a healthcare professional*: Before starting any fasting regimen, consult with your healthcare provider to ensure it's safe and suitable for your specific health needs.

2. *Choose a suitable fasting method*: Consider options like the 16/8 method (16 hours of fasting, 8 hours of eating) or the 5:2 method (eating normally for 5 days and restricting calories on 2 non-consecutive days). Find a method that aligns with your lifestyle.

3. *Monitor blood sugar levels*: Keep a close eye on your blood sugar levels during fasting to make adjustments as needed. Frequent monitoring helps prevent extreme highs or lows.

4. *Balanced diet during eating windows*: Focus on nutrient-dense foods, including lean proteins, whole grains, vegetables, and healthy fats, to support blood sugar control.

5. *Stay hydrated*: Drink plenty of water throughout the fasting period to avoid dehydration and help control hunger.

6. *Avoid excessive calorie restriction*: Don't cut calories too drastically; aim for a sustainable calorie deficit to avoid muscle loss and metabolic slowdown.

7. *Gradual adjustments*: If you're new to intermittent fasting, start with shorter fasting periods and gradually increase the duration as your body adapts.

8. *Medication adjustments*: If you're taking diabetes medications, consult your healthcare provider to adjust dosages as needed when implementing fasting.

9. *Prioritize sleep*: Ensure you get adequate sleep as it plays a significant role in blood sugar regulation.

10. *Listen to your body*: Pay attention to how your body responds to fasting. If you experience adverse effects, such as dizziness or extreme hunger, consider modifying your fasting schedule.

11. *Support network*: Share your fasting plan with friends or family, or consider joining a support group for motivation and accountability.

12. *Regular check-ups*: Continue to see your healthcare provider regularly for diabetes management and adjustments to your fasting plan, if necessary.

Remember that intermittent fasting may not be suitable for everyone with type 2 diabetes, and individual responses can vary. Always prioritize your health and safety by working closely with your healthcare team when implementing any fasting regimen.

Chapter 6

Safety Considerations and Precautions

Safety considerations and precautions are the ideas and steps you take to keep yourself safe while performing an action. It's similar to utilizing safety equipment while playing sports to prevent injury or wearing a seatbelt while driving to prevent harm in case of an accident. It refers to being cautious and taking precautions to make sure that intermittent fasting doesn't impair your health. This includes speaking with a healthcare provider, drinking plenty of water, eating healthfully when you're hungry, and paying attention to your body's cues to keep away from any potential hazards or pain. It basically involves looking after yourself while trying something new.

When embarking on an intermittent fasting journey, it's crucial to prioritize safety and take necessary precautions. Here are some key safety considerations:

- Consult with a Healthcare Professional

Before starting any fasting regimen, especially if you have underlying medical conditions, it's essential to consult with a healthcare provider. They can provide personalized guidance and ensure fasting is safe for you.

- Stay Hydrated

Dehydration can be a concern during fasting periods. Drink plenty of water throughout the fasting window to stay hydrated. Herbal teas and black coffee (without added sugar or cream) are also usually acceptable in moderation.

- Balanced Nutrition

During eating windows, focus on nutrient-dense foods to ensure you're getting essential vitamins and minerals. Incorporate fruits, vegetables, lean proteins, and whole grains into your meals.

- Avoid Overeating

It's tempting to indulge during eating windows, but overeating can negate the benefits of fasting. Practice mindful eating, and pay attention to portion sizes.

- Monitor Your Body

Listen to your body's signals. If you experience extreme hunger, dizziness, nausea, or other discomfort, consider adjusting your fasting schedule or breaking the fast.

- Medications and Health Conditions

If you take medications, especially those that require food, discuss your fasting plans with your healthcare provider. Some medical conditions may not be compatible with certain fasting methods.

- Gradual Adaptation

If you're new to fasting, start gradually. Begin with shorter fasting periods and gradually increase the duration as your body adjusts.

- Pregnancy and Breastfeeding

Intermittent fasting is generally not recommended for pregnant or breastfeeding women, as they have increased nutritional requirements. Consult with a healthcare professional for guidance.

- Avoid Extreme Fasts

Extended fasts lasting several days should only be attempted under medical supervision. These can carry risks and should not be done without careful consideration.

- Monitor Progress

Keep track of your progress and how you feel throughout your fasting journey. If you notice any adverse effects on your health or well-being, consult with a healthcare provider and consider adjusting your approach.

Keep in mind that intermittent fasting isn't a universal solution, and there's no single method that works for everyone. Your safety should be the top priority, so it's crucial to customize your fasting plan to suit your unique situation. When done sensibly and under expert advice, intermittent fasting can provide numerous health advantages.

Potential Risks and Side Effects

Intermittent fasting, like any dietary strategy, can have potential risks and side effects. It's essential to be aware of these before starting an intermittent fasting regimen:

1. Hunger and Irritability: Fasting periods can lead to hunger and irritability, which may be challenging to manage, especially initially.

2. Nutrient Deficiency: If not done carefully, intermittent fasting can result in nutrient deficiencies if you don't get enough essential vitamins and minerals during eating windows.

3. Fatigue and Weakness: Some individuals may experience fatigue, weakness, or low energy levels, particularly during extended fasting periods.

4. Headaches: Dehydration or changes in blood sugar levels during fasting can lead to headaches.

5. Dizziness and Lightheadedness: Fasting can cause dizziness or lightheadedness, especially when transitioning from sitting or lying down to standing.

6. Gastrointestinal Issues: Some people may experience digestive problems like constipation or acid reflux when changing eating patterns.

7. Loss of Muscle Mass: Prolonged fasting without proper protein intake can lead to muscle loss.

8. Disordered Eating: For some individuals, intermittent fasting can trigger or exacerbate disordered eating patterns.

9. Social Challenges: Fasting can make social situations, such as meals with friends and family, more complicated.

10. Not Suitable for Everyone: As mentioned earlier, certain groups of people, such as pregnant or nursing women and those with certain medical conditions, should avoid or carefully consider intermittent fasting.

Before beginning an intermittent fasting strategy, it is essential to speak with a healthcare provider or certified dietitian in order to reduce these dangers. They can assist you in developing a strategy that is fit for your requirements and goals and is safe. Additionally, pay attention to your body, drink enough water, and make sure you continue to eat a healthy, balanced meal throughout your eating windows.

Chapter 7

The Benefits of Intermittent Fasting for Women with Type 2 Diabetes

Think of intermittent fasting as a strong ally for women with Type 2 Diabetes, a top-secret tool that can help them control their weight, better regulate their blood sugar, enhance their general health, balance their hormones, and even improve their mood and cognitive abilities. It resembles having a complex tool in your toolbox for managing diabetes. However, it's essential to speak with a medical expert before starting this trip to make sure it fits with your unique health requirements and goals. With the appropriate direction, intermittent fasting can be a superhero in your diabetes management tale.

Intermittent fasting can offer several potential benefits for women with type 2 diabetes:

1. Weight Management and Body Composition

Unquestionably, regulating one's weight and body composition is essential for managing type 2 diabetes. By assisting people in controlling their calorie intake, intermittent fasting may be a helpful technique in reaching this objective. A calorie deficit, which is necessary for weight loss or maintaining a healthy weight, can be produced by limiting eating to specified time windows or decreasing the frequency of meals. The management of type 2 diabetes may then be enhanced by improving insulin sensitivity. However, it's crucial to approach intermittent fasting under the direction of a healthcare provider, especially for those with diabetes, to make sure it fits with their unique health needs and objectives.

2. Improved Blood Sugar Control

For people with type 2 diabetes, intermittent fasting can indeed help them control their blood sugar levels. Fasting can improve insulin sensitivity, which improves the body's ability to use insulin to control blood sugar levels. This increased insulin sensitivity can result in blood sugar levels that are more consistent and manageable, which is essential for treating diabetes. In order to make sure that intermittent fasting is a safe and effective strategy for their unique needs, diabetics must regularly monitor their blood sugar levels and collaborate with their healthcare team.

3. Enhancing Overall Health

Intermittent fasting has the potential to offer additional benefits for individuals with diabetes:

- Cellular Repair: During fasting periods, cells may undergo a process called autophagy, which involves the removal of damaged components. This cellular repair process can be particularly beneficial for overall health, including those with diabetes.

- Reduced Inflammation: Fasting has been linked to a reduction in inflammatory markers in some studies. Since inflammation plays a role in diabetes complications, this can be advantageous for managing the condition.

- Heart Health: Intermittent fasting may support cardiovascular health by reducing risk factors like high blood pressure and improving cholesterol levels. This is important for individuals with diabetes, as they are at higher risk for heart-related issues.

Although intermittent fasting appears promising, different people may react differently to it. Therefore, it is crucial to get medical advice to verify that intermittent fasting is secure and suitable for a person's unique health situation and requirements, particularly for people with diabetes.

4. Impact on Hormonal Balance and PCOS Management

Fasting may have a positive impact on hormonal balance, and this can be particularly relevant for women with polycystic ovary syndrome (PCOS). PCOS is often associated with insulin resistance, which can contribute to hormonal imbalances and other health issues, including an increased risk of type 2 diabetes.

Intermittent fasting has been studied as a potential strategy to improve insulin sensitivity, which can help regulate hormones in women with PCOS. By enhancing insulin sensitivity, fasting may contribute to better hormonal balance and potentially alleviate some PCOS symptoms.

However, it's crucial for women with PCOS to approach fasting under the guidance of a healthcare provider or registered dietitian who can provide personalized recommendations, as PCOS can vary widely in its presentation, and individual needs may differ. It's important to ensure that any fasting regimen is safe and appropriate for an individual's specific health condition and goals.

5. Cognitive Benefits and Mood

Some studies have suggested that intermittent fasting may have cognitive benefits and potentially improve mood, which can have a positive impact on the daily life of individuals with diabetes:

- Cognitive Benefits: Intermittent fasting might promote brain health by supporting processes like neuroplasticity and the production of brain-derived neurotrophic factor (BDNF). These mechanisms could potentially enhance cognitive function, memory, and overall brain health.

- Mood Improvement: Fasting can influence various hormones and neurotransmitters that play a role in mood regulation. Some individuals may experience improved mood and reduced symptoms of conditions like depression or anxiety as a result of intermittent fasting.

Although these possible advantages for mood and cognition are intriguing, it's important to keep in mind that different people will react differently to fasting.

Additionally, it is crucial for people with diabetes to keep their blood sugar levels steady. Therefore, it is important to proceed with any fasting regimen cautiously and in cooperation with a healthcare professional to make sure that it is compatible with the individual's unique health requirements and diabetes management strategy.

Chapter 8

The Future of Intermittent Fasting and Diabetes Management

The Future of Intermittent Fasting and Diabetes Management, refers to what we can expect to see in the coming years regarding how intermittent fasting is used to help manage diabetes. Think of it as a sneak peek into the potential changes, breakthroughs, and exciting developments in how we approach diabetes care with intermittent fasting. This includes things like personalized fasting plans, cutting-edge research, and the use of technology like wearables and apps, and even new ways to combine fasting with other treatments for better results.

It's all about making diabetes management more effective and tailored to each person's needs.

Ongoing Research and Innovations

Research and innovations related to the future of intermittent fasting (IF) in diabetes management continue to evolve.

Here are some ongoing areas of interest and exploration:

1. Effectiveness and Safety: The long-term efficacy and safety of different intermittent fasting protocols for people with diabetes are the subject of ongoing research. This includes studies examining various fasting lengths, frequency, and meal intervals to identify the most advantageous strategies.

2. Mechanisms of Action: In-depth investigations into the cellular and molecular mechanisms underpinning how intermittent fasting affects insulin sensitivity, blood sugar control, and general metabolic health are now being conducted. More specialized interventions may result from this understanding.

3. Individualized Approaches: Personalized medicine is gaining prominence, and researchers are investigating how to tailor intermittent fasting regimens based on an individual's genetics, metabolic profile, and response to fasting.

4. Technological Integration: Fasting schedules are being incorporated with improvements in wearable health technology and continuous glucose monitoring (CGM). For diabetics, fasting times and insulin dosages can be optimized using clever algorithms that use real-time glucose data.

5. Gut Microbiome Research: Studies are still being conducted to better understand how the gut microbiota affects diabetes and how intermittent fasting may affect gut

health. This study may result in treatments that enhance the microbiota for better blood sugar regulation.

6. Combination Therapies: Researchers are looking into how intermittent fasting might work in conjunction with other diabetes care techniques, such as prescription drugs, nutritional supplements, or lifestyle changes.

7. Psychological and Behavioral Aspects: Understanding the psychological and behavioral factors that influence adherence to fasting regimens is a growing area of research. Strategies to support behavior change and long-term adherence are being developed.

8. Telehealth and Remote Monitoring: The management of diabetes is being advanced by the integration of telehealth and remote monitoring. By giving patients real-time data and assistance, enabling improved adherence and individualized care plans, researchers are investigating how these technologies can improve the implementation and monitoring of intermittent fasting. Improved health outcomes and more effective diabetes treatment may result from this.

9. Prevention Focus: Some studies are exploring the role of intermittent fasting in diabetes prevention, especially among individuals at high risk of developing type 2 diabetes. This preventive approach may have significant public health implications.

10. Health Disparities: Researchers are working to address health disparities in diabetes management, including how intermittent fasting strategies can be made more accessible and culturally sensitive to diverse populations.

11. Collaborative Efforts: The world's researchers are working together more and more to exchange information and analysis on intermittent fasting and diabetes. Such teamwork can hasten the process and produce more reliable results.

12. Regulatory Considerations: Regulators may create policies and suggestions for the safe and efficient use of intermittent fasting in the treatment of diabetes as it grows in popularity.

Overall, the current research and advances in the field of managing diabetes with intermittent fasting are diverse and dynamic. They seek to improve the efficacy, security, and customization of fasting regimes, thereby enhancing the quality of life and health outcomes for people with diabetes.

Potential Breakthroughs

Imagine a future where managing diabetes is as personalized as choosing your favorite playlist. Breakthroughs in diabetes management are bringing us closer to this reality. Picture this: tailored fasting plans, like a customized diet playlist, designed specifically for your unique needs. Smart devices that keep an eye on your blood sugar in real-time, ensuring you stay in the diabetes management groove. Virtual fasting coaches to motivate and guide you through the process, accessible from the comfort of your home. Plus, AI wizards predicting your body's fasting dance moves and wearable tech adding a dash of style to your diabetes care routine.

It's not just about managing diabetes; it's about making it as smooth and enjoyable as your favorite tunes." The future of diabetes management, including the role of intermittent fasting, may witness several potential breakthroughs:

1. Precision Medicine: Advances in genetics and personalized medicine could lead to tailored diabetes treatments, including fasting regimens, based on an individual's genetic and metabolic profile. This approach may optimize the effectiveness of interventions.

2. Artificial Intelligence (AI) and Predictive Analytics: AI-driven algorithms could analyze vast amounts of health data to predict glucose fluctuations and recommend fasting schedules or dietary choices in real-time, enhancing diabetes control.

3. Innovative Medications: Ongoing research may yield novel medications that complement intermittent fasting, improving insulin sensitivity and glucose regulation with fewer side effects.

4. Continuous Glucose Monitoring (CGM) Enhancements: CGM technology could become more sophisticated, offering closed-loop systems that automatically adjust insulin delivery or recommend fasting strategies based on real-time glucose data.

5. Immunotherapy for Type 1 Diabetes: Immunotherapies that target the autoimmune response responsible for type 1 diabetes may become more effective, potentially reducing or eliminating the need for insulin therapy.

6. Gut Microbiome Manipulation: Emerging research on the gut microbiome's influence on metabolic health may lead to interventions that optimize gut bacteria for better blood sugar control, potentially in synergy with fasting.

7. Advanced Wearable Devices: Wearable health tech could evolve to provide more comprehensive health monitoring, including markers related to diabetes, helping individuals better understand and manage their condition.

8. Regenerative Medicine: Regenerative therapies, such as stem cell treatments, could offer new possibilities for repairing damaged pancreatic cells in type 1 diabetes or improving insulin production in type 2 diabetes.

9. Behavioral Health Integration: Comprehensive diabetes care may incorporate more robust psychological and behavioral support to address the emotional and lifestyle factors impacting diabetes management.

10. Telemedicine and Remote Monitoring: The expansion of telehealth and remote monitoring may make it easier for individuals with diabetes to access expert care and receive real-time guidance on fasting and diabetes management.

11. Global Collaboration: International efforts in diabetes research and treatment strategies may lead to breakthroughs through collective knowledge sharing and collaboration.

It's important to note that while these potential breakthroughs are promising, they may take years or even decades to fully realize. In the meantime, individuals with diabetes should continue to work closely with healthcare providers to make informed choices about their diabetes management, including the incorporation of intermittent fasting where appropriate.

Empowering Women in Their Health Journey

Empowering women in their health journey is a crucial aspect of ensuring their overall well-being and addressing specific health concerns effectively. Here are some key considerations and strategies for empowering women in this regard:

1. Education and Awareness: Providing women with access to accurate and comprehensive health information is fundamental. This includes information about nutrition, exercise, preventive care, reproductive health, and chronic

disease management. Education empowers women to make informed decisions about their health.

2. Regular Checkups and Screenings: Encourage women to prioritize regular health checkups and screenings. Healthcare providers can detect and address health issues early, which often leads to better outcomes. Empower women to be proactive in seeking preventive care.

3. Promoting a Holistic Approach: Emphasize the importance of a holistic approach to health, considering physical, mental, and emotional well-being. Encourage self-care practices like stress management, meditation, and mindfulness.

4. Nutrition and Healthy Eating: Educate women about the role of nutrition in health and disease prevention. Provide resources and support for adopting balanced and sustainable dietary habits that meet their unique nutritional needs.

5. Physical Activity: Promote regular physical activity and exercise, tailored to individual preferences and abilities. Physical fitness contributes to overall health, reduces the risk of chronic diseases, and enhances well-being.

6. Mental Health Support: Addressing mental health is vital. Create safe spaces for women to discuss their mental health concerns, reduce stigma, and provide access to mental health resources and professionals.

7. Reproductive Health Choices: Respect women's autonomy in making reproductive health choices. Provide comprehensive family planning options, prenatal and postnatal care, and support for fertility issues.

8. Chronic Disease Management: For women living with chronic conditions like diabetes, offer personalized care plans and resources. Encourage active involvement in managing their conditions and seeking regular medical guidance.

9. Support Networks: Foster supportive communities where women can share experiences, seek advice, and find encouragement. Support groups can be invaluable for those dealing with specific health challenges.

10. Access to Healthcare: Ensure that women have equitable access to healthcare services, including contraception, maternal care, and treatment for chronic diseases. Address barriers such as affordability, transportation, and cultural sensitivity.

11. Advocacy and Representation: Encourage women to become advocates for their own health and participate in decision-making processes related to healthcare policies and research. Representation of women's health needs is vital in shaping healthcare systems.

12. Cultural Sensitivity: Recognize and respect diverse cultural beliefs and practices related to health. Tailor healthcare interventions to be culturally sensitive and inclusive.

In addition to promoting personal wellbeing, empowering women in their pursuit of good health is a step toward attaining gender equality in healthcare. We can assist women in taking charge of their health and leading better, more satisfying lives by giving them the tools, knowledge, and support they need.

Chapter 9

FAQs and Common Concerns

Here are some frequently asked questions and common concerns about intermittent fasting for women with type 2 diabetes:

1. *Is intermittent fasting safe for women with type 2 diabetes?*

- Intermittent fasting can be safe for women with type 2 diabetes, but it should be approached cautiously and under the guidance of a healthcare professional.

2. *What are the potential benefits of intermittent fasting for women with type 2 diabetes?*

- Intermittent fasting may help improve insulin sensitivity, aid in weight loss, and better blood sugar control.

3. *What is the best fasting schedule for women with type 2 diabetes?*

- The ideal fasting schedule varies from person to person. Common approaches include the 16/8 method (16 hours fasting, 8-hour eating window) or the 5:2 method (eating normally for 5 days and restricting calories for 2 days).

Consult with a healthcare provider to determine the best plan.

4. *Can intermittent fasting lead to low blood sugar (hypoglycemia) in women with diabetes?*

- It's possible, so careful monitoring of blood sugar levels is crucial. Adjustments to medications and meal timing may be necessary.

5. *Should women with type 2 diabetes avoid fasting during their menstrual cycle?*

- Some women may find fasting more challenging during their menstrual cycle due to hormonal fluctuations. It's a personal choice and can be adjusted as needed.

6. *What should I eat during the eating window when practicing intermittent fasting?*

- Choose nutrient-dense foods like lean proteins, whole grains, fruits, vegetables, and healthy fats to support stable blood sugar levels.

7. *Is it safe to exercise during fasting periods for women with type 2 diabetes?*

- Exercise can be beneficial, but it's essential to monitor blood sugar levels and adjust workouts accordingly. Low-intensity activities may be safer during fasting.

8. *Can intermittent fasting be used as a long-term strategy for managing type 2 diabetes in women?*

- Long-term fasting should be discussed with a healthcare provider. It may not be suitable for everyone, and individualized plans are essential.

9. *What are the signs that intermittent fasting isn't working for me?*

- If you experience persistent low blood sugar, extreme hunger, fatigue, or other adverse effects, it's essential to consult with your healthcare provider and consider alternative strategies.

10. *Are there any specific supplements or vitamins that can support women with type 2 diabetes during intermittent fasting?*

- Supplements like magnesium and chromium may help, but always consult with a healthcare provider before adding any supplements to your regimen.

11. *Is it safe to fast if I'm pregnant or breastfeeding and have type 2 diabetes?*

- Fasting during pregnancy or while breastfeeding is generally not recommended, as it's crucial to provide adequate nutrients for both you and your baby. Consult with a healthcare provider for guidance.

12. *Can intermittent fasting help with weight loss for women with type 2 diabetes?*

- Intermittent fasting can aid in weight loss, but it's essential to focus on overall diet quality and consult with a healthcare provider to ensure it aligns with your diabetes management plan.

13. *Are there any potential side effects of intermittent fasting for women with type 2 diabetes?*

- Side effects can include irritability, hunger, and difficulty concentrating. However, these are often temporary and can be managed with adjustments to your fasting schedule and diet.

14. *Can I drink water or other beverages during the fasting period?*

- Yes, staying hydrated is essential. You can drink water, herbal tea, or other non-caloric beverages during the fasting period. However, avoid sugary drinks and excessive caffeine.

15. *Should I check my blood sugar more frequently while fasting?*

- Yes, monitoring your blood sugar levels is crucial during fasting to ensure they stay within a safe range. Follow your healthcare provider's recommendations for testing frequency.

16. *What is the "dawn phenomenon," and how does it relate to fasting for women with type 2 diabetes?*

- The dawn phenomenon refers to a natural increase in blood sugar levels in the early morning hours. Fasting can sometimes exacerbate this effect, so it's essential to work with your healthcare provider to manage it effectively.

17. *Can intermittent fasting be combined with other dietary approaches, like a low-carb or Mediterranean diet?*

- Yes, combining intermittent fasting with other dietary strategies can be effective. Discuss with your healthcare provider to create a comprehensive plan that suits your needs.

18. *How long does it take to see improvements in blood sugar control with intermittent fasting?*

- The time it takes to see improvements can vary from person to person. Some individuals may notice changes within a few weeks, while others may take longer. Consistency is key.

19. *Are there any special considerations for women with type 2 diabetes who have a history of eating disorders?*

- Women with a history of eating disorders should approach fasting cautiously, if at all, and only under the guidance of a healthcare provider who specializes in eating disorders.

20. What resources or support networks are available for women with type 2 diabetes interested in trying intermittent fasting?

- Consider seeking guidance from registered dietitians, diabetes educators, or support groups specific to diabetes management and intermittent fasting. They can provide valuable information and support.

Recognize that managing type 2 diabetes with intermittent fasting requires a highly individualized approach. Since everyone's response to intermittent fasting is unique, it's important to create a schedule that fits your specific requirements and health goals.

Before making major adjustments to your fasting schedule or diabetes treatment strategy, always speak with your healthcare professional.

Addressing Common Questions and Misconceptions

Let's clear up some frequent misunderstandings and issues about intermittent fasting for type 2 diabetic women:

1. *Misconception*: Intermittent fasting is a one-size-fits-all approach.

- *Fact*: Intermittent fasting should be personalized. What works for one person may not work for another. Factors like age, activity level, and diabetes management goals should be considered when designing a fasting plan.

2. *Misconception*: Fasting means skipping meals and starving oneself.

- *Fact*: Fasting involves controlled periods of not eating, but it doesn't mean starving. Properly planned fasting schedules aim to optimize nutrient intake during eating windows.

3. *Misconception*: Intermittent fasting will cure type 2 diabetes.

- *Fact*: While intermittent fasting can help manage blood sugar levels and improve insulin sensitivity, it's not a cure for type 2 diabetes. Diabetes management often requires a comprehensive approach that may include medication, diet, and lifestyle changes.

4. *Misconception*: Fasting leads to muscle loss.

- *Fact*: Intermittent fasting, when done correctly, should not result in significant muscle loss. Maintaining an adequate protein intake during eating windows can help preserve muscle mass.

5. *Misconception*: Fasting causes extreme hunger and binge eating.

- *Fact*: Fasting can cause increased hunger initially, but this often stabilizes over time. Planning balanced, nutritious meals during eating windows can help prevent binge eating.

6. *Misconception*: Women with type 2 diabetes should always avoid fasting.**

- *Fact*: Fasting can be safe and beneficial for some women with type 2 diabetes when done under medical supervision and with careful planning. It's not a one-size-fits-all recommendation, and individualized guidance is essential.

7. *Misconception*: Fasting must follow a strict schedule.

- *Fact*: Fasting schedules can be flexible. Some days may require longer fasts, while others can be shorter. Flexibility allows adaptation to individual needs and lifestyles.

8. *Misconception*: Fasting is only about weight loss.

- *Fact*: While weight loss can be a result of intermittent fasting, it offers other health benefits, such as improved insulin sensitivity, reduced inflammation, and potential longevity benefits.

9. *Misconception*: Intermittent fasting is unsafe for women during menopause.

- *Fact*: Menopausal women can engage in intermittent fasting, but hormonal changes may affect how they respond. Consultation with a healthcare provider can help tailor a fasting plan.

10. *Misconception*: Intermittent fasting is a quick fix for diabetes management.

- *Fact*: Managing type 2 diabetes requires long-term commitment. Intermittent fasting can be a tool in your diabetes management toolbox but should be combined with other strategies for optimal results.

11. *Misconception*: Fasting will lead to nutrient deficiencies.

- *Fact*: Properly planned intermittent fasting allows for nutrient-rich meals during eating windows, reducing the risk of deficiencies. Monitoring your diet is essential to ensure adequate nutrition.

12. *Misconception*: It's necessary to skip breakfast to practice intermittent fasting.

- *Fact*: Intermittent fasting doesn't mandate skipping breakfast. You can choose an eating window that aligns with your daily routine and preferences, whether it starts with breakfast or later in the day.

13. *Misconception*: Fasting causes a drop in metabolism.

* *Fact*: Short-term fasting may have a minimal impact on metabolism, and it's usually compensated for by increased fat oxidation. Long-term effects on metabolism are still a subject of research.

14. *Misconception*: You should fast every day to see benefits.

* *Fact*: You don't need to fast daily. Many people find success with intermittent fasting by doing it a few times a week or even less frequently, depending on their goals.

15. *Misconception*: Fasting is too difficult to maintain in the long run.

* *Fact*: Fasting can become a sustainable part of your lifestyle with practice and adaptation. Over time, your body may adjust, and fasting can become easier.

16. *Misconception*: Intermittent fasting is unsafe for older women with type 2 diabetes.

* *Fact*: Older women can safely practice intermittent fasting, but they may need to tailor their fasting plan to their specific health needs and limitations. Consultation with a healthcare provider is advisable.

17. *Misconception*: You must eat specific foods during your eating window.

- *Fact*: There is no one-size-fits-all approach to what you should eat during your eating window. Focus on balanced, nutritious meals that align with your dietary preferences and diabetes management goals.

18. *Misconception*: Fasting is a replacement for diabetes medication.

- *Fact*: Fasting should not be used as a sole replacement for prescribed diabetes medication. Medication adjustments should be made under the guidance of a healthcare provider when fasting is introduced.

19. *Misconception*: Fasting leads to a decline in energy levels.

- *Fact*: Some individuals may experience a temporary dip in energy during fasting, but others report increased mental clarity and energy once their bodies adapt to the routine.

20. *Misconception*: You should ignore your body's hunger cues during fasting.

- *Fact*: Ignoring extreme hunger signals during fasting can be counterproductive. It's essential to listen to your body and make adjustments to your fasting schedule or meal composition if needed.

Remember that intermittent fasting can be an effective tool for managing type 2 diabetes, but it's crucial to take a fair and informed stance when using it. Making the most of this nutritional strategy safely and efficiently requires working with a healthcare professional and paying close attention to your body's reaction.

Conclusion

It's important to approach this dietary strategy for women with type 2 diabetes in the context of intermittent fasting with a fair and informed viewpoint. Improved insulin sensitivity, better blood sugar regulation, and potential weight loss are just a few advantages of intermittent fasting. The best way to achieve these benefits is to be led by fundamental ideas and have a clear grasp of how this plan fits into a larger health strategy.

Key Takeaways

Personalization comes first and is crucial. There is no one-size-fits-all method of intermittent fasting. Every woman has different daily habits, interests, and health requirements. Therefore, it's essential to customize intermittent fasting strategies in accordance with individual needs and health objectives.

The key to successful intermittent fasting is still nutrition. To avoid vitamin deficiency and enhance general wellbeing, it is crucial to ensure balanced, nutrient-rich meals during eating windows. Nutritional needs are not sacrificed by fasting. It's also critical to stress that intermittent fasting is not a quick answer. It requires a lengthy commitment. While it can be a useful tool for managing diabetes, it should be viewed as part of a comprehensive plan that also includes elements like medicine, exercise, and routine blood sugar monitoring.

Your Next Steps

The following actions are obvious for ladies who are thinking about intermittent fasting. Consult a healthcare practitioner with experience in diabetes management to get started. They can work with you to develop a customized fasting strategy that supports your unique health goals and offer advice on how to carry it out safely. Another crucial component of the path is educational empowerment. To make wise decisions regarding your health, keep studying about managing diabetes, diet, and various fasting methods.

The next steps are simple for ladies who are thinking about intermittent fasting. Consult a healthcare practitioner who is knowledgeable in diabetes management to start. They can offer advice on how to safely carry out your customized fasting plan, which will be in line with your unique health goals.
Another crucial component of the path is empowerment through education. To make wise decisions regarding your health, keep studying about diet, managing your diabetes, and different fasting methods.

Finally, keep in mind that dedication is essential to managing diabetes. It is an ongoing journey. As you negotiate the challenges and successes of intermittent fasting, stay committed to your health goals and have patience with yourself.

Empowering Women to Take Control of Their Health

With education and encouragement, empowerment may start. Women can take charge of their health and improve their quality of life by adopting a holistic approach to managing their diabetes, which includes intermittent fasting as a useful tool. Bettering one's general health and blood sugar control is a goal that is not simply aspirational but also doable.

Recognize that you have the power to make improvements to your health. You can successfully manage type 2 diabetes while leading a fulfilling and health-conscious lifestyle with the correct advice and unwavering resolve. Intermittent fasting can be a significant component of your journey to a healthier and happier life. Your health journey is yours to define and direct.

References

https://healthmatch.io/type-2-diabetes/signs-of-type-2-diabetes-in-women

https://my.clevelandclinic.org/health/diseases/21501-type-2-diabetes

https://pubmed.ncbi.nlm.nih.gov/36897358/

https://www.carbmanager.com/article/yoherxeaaceazayu/how-to-choose-an-intermittent-fasting-schedule

https://www.cdc.gov/diabetes/basics/type2.html

https://www.diabetesfoodhub.org/articles/what-is-a-low-carb-diet.html

https://www.freepik.com/free-photo/blue-alarm-clock-white-background_903337.htm#

https://www.freepik.com/free-photo/portrait-young-businesswoman-holding-eyeglasses-hand-against-graybackdrop_3717378.htm#

https://www.healthline.com/nutrition/improve-insulin-sensitivity#

https://www.healthline.com/nutrition/insulin-and-insulin-resistance#

https://www.healthline.com/nutrition/intermittent-fasting-guide

https://www.medicalnewstoday.com/articles/diabetes-affects-men-women#treatment

https://www.ncbi.nlm.nih.gov/pmc/articles/PMC10163139/

https://www.ncbi.nlm.nih.gov/pmc/articles/PMC7310804/

https://www.ncbi.nlm.nih.gov/pmc/articles/PMC8360708/

https://www.niddk.nih.gov/health-
    information/diabetes/overview/what-is-diabetes/type-2-
    diabetes
https://www.webmd.com/diabetes/type-2-diabetes
https://www.who.int/news-room/fact-sheets/detail/diabetes

www.ingramcontent.com/pod-product-compliance
Lightning Source LLC
Chambersburg PA
CBHW060747260726
48660CB00002B/519